Dry Fasting

A Beginner's Quick Start Overview on Its Use Cases, With a Potential 5-Step Plan

mf

copyright © 2024 Stephanie Hinderock

All rights reserved No part of this book may be reproduced, or stored in a retrieval system, or transmitted in any form or by any means, electronic, mechanical, photocopying, recording, or otherwise, without express written permission of the publisher.

Disclaimer

By reading this disclaimer, you are accepting the terms of the disclaimer in full. If you disagree with this disclaimer, please do not read the guide.

All of the content within this guide is provided for informational and educational purposes only, and should not be accepted as independent medical or other professional advice. The author is not a doctor, physician, nurse, mental health provider, or registered nutritionist/dietician. Therefore, using and reading this guide does not establish any form of a physician-patient relationship.

Always consult with a physician or another qualified health provider with any issues or questions you might have regarding any sort of medical condition. Do not ever disregard any qualified professional medical advice or delay seeking that advice because of anything you have read in this guide. The information in this guide is not intended to be any sort of medical advice and should not be used in lieu of any medical advice by a licensed and qualified medical professional.

The information in this guide has been compiled from a variety of known sources. However, the author cannot attest to or guarantee the accuracy of each source and thus should not be held liable for any errors or omissions.

You acknowledge that the publisher of this guide will not be held liable for any loss or damage of any kind incurred as a result of this guide or the reliance on any information provided within this guide. You acknowledge and agree that you assume all risk and responsibility for any action you undertake in response to the information in this guide.

Using this guide does not guarantee any particular result (e.g., weight loss or a cure). By reading this guide, you acknowledge that there are no guarantees to any specific outcome or results you can expect.

All product names, diet plans, or names used in this guide are for identification purposes only and are the property of their respective owners. The use of these names does not imply endorsement. All other trademarks cited herein are the property of their respective owners.

Where applicable, this guide is not intended to be a substitute for the original work of this diet plan and is, at most, a supplement to the original work for this diet plan and never a direct substitute. This guide is a personal expression of the facts of that diet plan.

Where applicable, persons shown in the cover images are stock photography models and the publisher has obtained the rights to use the images through license agreements with third-party stock image companies.

Table of Contents

Introduction   6
What Is Dry Fasting?   8
   Types of Dry Fasting   8
   How Dry Fasting Affects the Body   10
   Use Cases of Dry Fasting   11
   Is Dry Fasting Right For You?   13
Comparison of Fasting Types   16
   Understanding Water Fasting and Intermittent Fasting   16
   Key Differences Between Dry Fasting and Other Fasting Methods   17
   Hydration and Food Intake   17
   Metabolic Effects   20
   Duration and Intensity   24
   Outcomes and Experiences   28
   Pros and Cons of Dry Fasting   30
   Risk and Precautions   33
Potential Benefits of Dry Fasting   37
   Physical Health Benefits   37
   Mental and Emotional Benefits   39
5-Step Plan to Getting Started with Dry Fasting   41
   Step 1: Research and Education about Dry Fasting   41
   Step 2: Consult with a Healthcare Provider for Personalized Advice   42
   Step 3: Start with Shorter Fasting Periods and Gradually Increase Duration   47
   Step 4: Implement Supportive Habits such as Proper Hydration Before and After Fasting   64
   Step 5: Monitor the Body's Response and Adjust the Approach as Necessary   68
Conclusion   73
FAQs   76
References and Helpful Links   78

Introduction

Dry fasting—a dietary practice that involves abstaining from both food and water—has been gaining attention in wellness circles for its purported health benefits. Unlike other fasting methods that allow fluids, dry fasting is known for its intensity and is believed to accelerate detoxification and healing processes in the body. However, as with many health trends, it is shrouded in controversy and is not universally endorsed by health professionals. Understanding the potential advantages, as well as the drawbacks, is crucial for anyone considering this practice.

In this guide you will learn about the following;

- What is Dry Fasting?
- Comparison of Fasting Types
- Potential Benefits of Dry Fasting
- How Does Dry Fasting Affect the Body
- Pros and Cons of Dry Fasting
- Risk and Precautions
- 5-Step Plan to Getting Started with Dry Fasting

This guide also provides a balanced view of its associated risks and offers a thoughtful five-step plan for those intrigued by the idea of starting a dry fast, all while maintaining an objective perspective to ensure informed decision-making. We do not recommend this practice as it may not be suitable for everyone.

Instead, our aim is to provide you with the necessary information so that you can make an informed decision about whether dry fasting is right for you. By the end of this guide, you will have a better understanding of what dry fasting entails and its potential use cases for health.

What Is Dry Fasting?

Dry fasting is the practice of abstaining from both food and water for a certain period of time. Unlike other types of fasting, such as water fasting or intermittent fasting, dry fasting restricts all forms of liquid consumption. This means that during a dry fast, no liquids are allowed including water, tea, coffee, or juices.

The origins of dry fasting can be traced back to ancient civilizations like Ancient Greece and Egypt. In these cultures, dry fasting was often practiced for spiritual and religious purposes. It was believed that by denying the body food and water, one could achieve greater mental clarity and spiritual enlightenment.

Types of Dry Fasting

There are two main types of dry fasting, each with its own set of guidelines and implications for health:

1. **Absolute (or Hard) Dry Fasting**

    This is the strictest form of dry fasting, where absolutely no contact with water is permitted. This means not only abstaining from drinking water, but also avoiding bathing, brushing teeth, or any other form of water contact.

This method is often practiced for shorter durations due to its intensity and can lead to significant physiological changes in the body. Because it completely eliminates hydration, meticulous planning is essential to avoid severe dehydration and other health complications.

2. **Soft Dry Fasting**

This approach allows for minimal contact with water, which can include activities like brushing your teeth or taking a quick shower. While this method still prohibits the consumption of any liquids, it offers a slightly more lenient framework compared to absolute dry fasting. Many individuals find this type more manageable, making it a popular choice for those new to fasting or those who may have concerns about hydration levels.

Both types of dry fasting require careful consideration and should be approached with caution due to the potential health risks involved. It's crucial to consult with a healthcare professional before attempting either method, especially for those with pre-existing medical conditions or concerns regarding their hydration status.

Understanding your body's needs and listening to its signals is key to safely navigating the fasting experience.

How Dry Fasting Affects the Body

Dry fasting initiates a profound series of physiological and biochemical adaptations, driving the body to optimize hydration, enhance cellular repair mechanisms, and strengthen immune resilience.

Physiological and Biochemical Effects

Dry fasting instigates a range of physiological and biochemical changes within the body. One of the most immediate effects is dehydration, which compels the body to optimize water utilization. During this state, hydration levels decrease, prompting the body to draw water internally through metabolic processes, such as the breakdown of fat.

Cellular repair mechanisms are also notably activated during dry fasting. The absence of external water and food intake triggers a survival response, driving the body to initiate autophagy—a process where cells degrade and recycle their own components. This not only aids in cellular repair but also enhances the elimination of damaged cells and toxins.

The immune response is another critical area affected by dry fasting. The stress induced by dehydration and nutrient scarcity can provoke a hormetic response, mild stress that stimulates protective processes in cells. This response can potentially enhance the body's resilience to stress and improve immune function over time.

Use Cases of Dry Fasting

Dry fasting serves a variety of purposes across different domains, particularly in health-related contexts, making it a multifaceted practice with distinct applications.

1. **Religious and Spiritual Practices:**

   In many religious traditions, dry fasting is a revered practice aimed at spiritual discipline and purification. It is often observed during holy seasons or specific religious events, such as Ramadan in Islam, where adherents fast from dawn until sunset.

   The absence of food and water during these times is seen as a way to purify the body and soul, fostering a deeper connection with the divine. This practice serves as a testament to one's faith, promoting self-control and reflection on spiritual values and beliefs.

2. **Cultural Traditions**

   Beyond religion, dry fasting is embedded in various cultural traditions and rituals. It is sometimes performed during festivals or ceremonies that mark significant life events or transitions. In these contexts, dry fasting is a means of paying homage to one's heritage and maintaining cultural identity. It acts as a communal practice that unites people, reinforcing shared values and cultural continuity across generations.

3. **Medical and Therapeutic Applications:**

   In the realm of alternative medicine, dry fasting is occasionally utilized as a therapeutic approach for certain health conditions. Practitioners may recommend it for its potential to stimulate autophagy and enhance detoxification processes.

   However, this use case requires careful consideration and should only be undertaken with the guidance of a healthcare professional, as the absence of water intake can pose risks if not properly managed.

4. **Mental and Emotional Challenges:**

   On an individual level, some people engage in dry fasting as a personal challenge to strengthen mental fortitude and self-discipline. The practice demands a high level of commitment and resilience, offering an opportunity for individuals to test their limits and enhance their ability to cope with stress. By voluntarily enduring the discomforts of fasting, individuals often report increased willpower and emotional stability, which can translate into other areas of life.

5. **Research and Study**

   From a scientific perspective, dry fasting is of interest to researchers studying its physiological effects and potential health impacts. Research in this area can provide insights into how the body adapts to extreme conditions and the potential benefits or risks associated with such practices. Additionally, anthropologists and sociologists may explore the cultural and religious significance of dry fasting, examining its role in shaping social and religious practices across different societies.

Overall, dry fasting continues to be a controversial and much-debated topic in the health and wellness world. While its benefits are not yet fully understood or scientifically proven, many people around the world continue to practice it for various reasons. As with any dietary or lifestyle change, it's essential to consult a healthcare professional before incorporating dry fasting into your routine.

Is Dry Fasting Right For You?

Determining if dry fasting is right for you involves considering several factors that can significantly impact your experience and outcomes. These include your current health status, lifestyle, and personal goals. Here are some key points to think about:

1. ***Health Status***: Your health is paramount when considering any fasting regimen. If you have chronic health conditions such as diabetes, heart disease, or any other medical issues, or if you are pregnant or breastfeeding, it is crucial to consult with a healthcare provider before attempting dry fasting. This ensures that you do not unintentionally jeopardize your health or that of your child. A medical professional can provide personalized advice based on your unique circumstances.

2. ***Experience with Fasting***: If you're new to fasting, it might be beneficial to start with less restrictive forms, like intermittent fasting, which allows you to eat during specific windows of the day. This approach helps you gauge how your body reacts to fasting without the challenges of completely abstaining from food and water. Gradually working your way up to dry fasting can help build your confidence and understanding of how your body responds to different fasting methods.

3. ***Goals***: Clearly defining what you hope to achieve with dry fasting is essential. Whether it's weight loss, enhanced mental clarity, or detoxification, having a specific target in mind will help you stay motivated. Additionally, it's important to assess if these goals align with your overall health strategy. For instance, if

weight loss is your primary goal, consider how dry fasting might complement your dietary choices and exercise routine for the best results.

4. **Lifestyle Compatibility**: Dry fasting requires careful planning and monitoring, which means you need to consider whether it fits into your daily routine and commitments. Evaluate your work schedule, social activities, and personal habits to determine if you can realistically integrate dry fasting into your life. If your lifestyle is busy with frequent meetings or social gatherings, it may be challenging to commit to a fasting schedule.

5. **Willingness to Monitor and Adjust**: Finally, be prepared to closely monitor your body's response to fasting and make necessary adjustments to your approach. Fasting can elicit various physical and emotional responses, and what's effective for one person may not work for another. Keeping a journal of your experiences can help you track changes in mood, energy levels, and physical health, allowing you to fine-tune your fasting strategy for optimal results.

By thoughtfully considering these factors, you can make a more informed decision about whether dry fasting is a suitable choice for you.

Comparison of Fasting Types

Fasting has become a popular strategy in the health and wellness community, with different types offering various benefits and challenges. Among these, dry fasting, water fasting, and intermittent fasting are three prominent methods. This chapter explores these fasting types, shedding light on their principles, differences, and typical outcomes.

Understanding Water Fasting and Intermittent Fasting

<u>Water Fasting</u> involves abstaining from all food while only consuming water. This fasting type is often chosen for its potential to detoxify the body, promote autophagy (the body's way of cleaning out damaged cells), and aid in weight loss. Water fasting can vary in duration, commonly ranging from 24 hours to several days, depending on the individual's experience and goals.

<u>Intermittent Fasting (IF)</u>, on the other hand, alternates between periods of eating and fasting. There are different methods of IF, such as the 16/8 method (fasting for 16 hours and eating during an 8-hour window) and the 5:2 approach

(eating regularly for five days and significantly reducing calorie intake for two non-consecutive days). Intermittent fasting is praised for its flexibility and its potential to improve metabolic health, enhance fat burning, and simplify dieting.

Key Differences Between Dry Fasting and Other Fasting Methods

Dry Fasting is more extreme as it prohibits all food and liquid intake, including water. It is based on the idea that the body can achieve a profound detoxification state when deprived of both nutrients and hydration. There are two types of dry fasting: *soft dry fasting*, where contact with water (like brushing teeth) is allowed, and *hard dry fasting*, where even skin contact with water is avoided.

Hydration and Food Intake

Fasting methods vary significantly in their approach to hydration and food intake, each offering unique benefits and challenges. Understanding these differences is crucial for anyone considering fasting as a health strategy.

1. **Dry Fasting: Total Fluid Restriction**
   - *Hydration Challenges*: Dry fasting involves abstaining from all fluids, including water. This complete restriction can lead to rapid dehydration, which can have several physiological effects such as decreased energy

levels, headaches, and dizziness. The lack of hydration requires the body to rely solely on its internal water reserves, which can accelerate detoxification processes but also increase the risk of dehydration-related complications.

- ***Potential Effects on the Body***: The absence of fluid intake forces the body into a more intense metabolic state. While some proponents believe this intensifies autophagy and fat metabolism, the risks of electrolyte imbalances and kidney strain must be carefully managed. Dry fasting is typically recommended for short durations and should be approached with caution, especially by those new to fasting.

2. **Water Fasting: Hydration through Water Intake**
   - ***Hydration Benefits***: Unlike dry fasting, water fasting permits the intake of water, which helps maintain hydration levels. This can make the fasting process more manageable and less taxing on the body, allowing for longer fasting periods compared to dry fasting.
   - ***Ease of Fasting Process***: Water supports basic metabolic functions and helps flush out toxins, making the fasting experience smoother. It can also alleviate some symptoms like hunger pangs, making it a more accessible option for

those looking to detoxify or reset their eating habits.

- *Challenges*: Despite allowing water, the absence of food can still lead to energy depletion and muscle loss if not carefully monitored. Extended water fasting should be done under supervision to prevent potential adverse effects on metabolism and overall health.

3. **Intermittent Fasting: Flexibility in Hydration and Nutrition**
    - *Hydration and Nutritional Balance*: Intermittent fasting is distinct in that it allows both eating and drinking within specific windows, offering greater flexibility in maintaining hydration and nutritional balance. This approach helps ensure that the body receives the necessary nutrients and fluids daily, reducing the risks associated with more restrictive fasting methods.

    - *Flexibility and Sustainability*: By structuring fasting around personal schedules, individuals can continue to enjoy social meals and maintain their usual hydration routines. This adaptability makes intermittent fasting a sustainable long-term practice for improving health and managing weight.

- ***Potential Challenges***: While intermittent fasting is generally less restrictive, it requires discipline to adhere to eating windows and to choose nutrient-dense foods. Balancing caloric intake and hydration within limited hours can be challenging, especially for those new to fasting.

In summary, each fasting method offers distinct approaches to hydration and food intake, influencing their effectiveness and suitability for different individuals. Dry fasting provides rapid detoxification but poses significant hydration challenges. Water fasting offers a more balanced approach with hydration support, while intermittent fasting combines nutritional flexibility with structured eating periods, making it a viable option for long-term health benefits.

Metabolic Effects

Fasting can significantly alter metabolic processes in the body, each method offering distinct pathways and outcomes. Here's a closer look at how dry fasting, water fasting, and intermittent fasting impact metabolism.

1. **Dry Fasting**
   - *Accelerated Autophagy*: Without water, dry fasting is believed to push the body into autophagy more rapidly. This process is crucial for cellular repair and detoxification, as old or damaged cells are broken down and recycled. The absence of water forces the body to rely more heavily on its internal resources, hastening this regenerative process.

   - *Increased Fat Metabolism*: Dry fasting encourages the body to enhance fat metabolism. Due to the lack of caloric intake and hydration, the body quickly turns to fat stores for energy, potentially leading to faster fat loss. This heightened metabolic activity can also aid in detoxifying the body, as fat cells often store toxins.

   - *Challenges*: The rigorous nature of dry fasting can be physically taxing, posing risks like dehydration and mineral loss if not managed carefully. This necessitates a cautious approach, typically suitable for those with previous fasting experience.

2. **Water Fasting**
   - *Gradual Autophagy*: Water fasting also promotes autophagy, albeit at a slower pace

compared to dry fasting. The presence of water allows the body to gradually enter a state of cellular cleanup, supporting detoxification and renewal over a more extended period.

- *Caloric Restriction*: By eliminating caloric intake, water fasting shifts metabolism towards utilizing stored energy, particularly fat. However, the transition may not be as rapid as in dry fasting due to the body's ongoing hydration.

- *Metabolic Impacts*: Extended water fasting can influence metabolism by reducing basal metabolic rate as the body attempts to conserve energy. This can pose a challenge, especially if fasting exceeds a few days without proper monitoring.

3. **Intermittent Fasting**
   - *Improved Insulin Sensitivity*: One of the most notable benefits of intermittent fasting is its impact on insulin sensitivity. By regularly reducing eating windows, the body becomes more efficient at managing blood glucose levels, reducing insulin resistance over time.

   - *Metabolic Flexibility*: Intermittent fasting enhances the body's ability to switch between burning carbohydrates and fats for energy, promoting metabolic flexibility. This adaptability can lead to sustained energy levels and improved overall metabolic health.

- ***Long-term Benefits***: Unlike more intense fasting methods, intermittent fasting can be seamlessly integrated into daily life, offering lasting benefits without extreme restrictions. However, the gradual nature of its metabolic effects requires consistent practice to achieve significant results.

Each fasting method uniquely influences metabolic processes. Dry fasting offers rapid benefits in autophagy and fat metabolism, with a need for careful management due to its intensity. Water fasting supports a slower yet steady metabolic transition, beneficial for detoxification but requiring monitoring over extended periods.

Intermittent fasting stands out for its sustainable impact on insulin sensitivity and metabolic flexibility, providing long-term advantages with consistent application. Understanding these effects helps individuals tailor their fasting practices to better align with their health goals.

Duration and Intensity

Fasting practices vary significantly in terms of duration and intensity, each offering unique benefits and challenges. Here's a detailed look at the differences between dry fasting, water fasting, and intermittent fasting, focusing on their typical durations and the reasons behind them.

1. **Dry Fasting**
    - *Duration*: Typically practiced for shorter periods, dry fasting usually ranges from 12 to 24 hours. This limited time frame helps to minimize potential negative effects on the body while still allowing for some of the benefits associated with fasting.

    - *Intensity*: Dry fasting is known for its heightened intensity due to the complete abstention from both food and water. This can lead to more pronounced physical and mental challenges, as the body must rely solely on its own reserves for energy and hydration during the fasting period.

    - *Risks*: The absence of water intake adds a significant level of difficulty and increases the risk of dehydration. Dehydration can lead to symptoms such as dizziness, headaches, and fatigue, which is why the fasting period is kept intentionally short to mitigate these risks. It is essential to listen to your body and recognize any signs of distress.

- ***Recommendation***: Dry fasting should be approached with caution and is best suited for those with prior fasting experience or under medical supervision. It's crucial for individuals to understand their own health conditions and limitations before engaging in this practice, as it may not be suitable for everyone, especially for those with underlying health issues.

2. **Water Fasting**
    - ***Duration***: A water fast can extend over several days, typically ranging from 24 hours to several weeks. The exact length often depends on the individual's overall health, previous fasting experience, and specific health objectives they aim to achieve. For instance, novice fasters may start with shorter durations to gauge their body's response, while more experienced individuals might undertake longer fasts for deeper detoxification or health benefits.
    - ***Intensity***: Water fasting is generally less intense than dry fasting because it allows for the consumption of water, which is crucial for maintaining hydration and supporting bodily

functions. This hydration can help mitigate some common side effects associated with fasting, such as headaches and fatigue, making the experience more manageable.

- *Factors Influencing Duration*: Several factors influence how long a person can safely engage in a water fast. The individual's health condition plays a critical role; those with underlying medical issues should approach fasting with caution and ideally under medical supervision. Additionally, a person's experience with fasting can affect their ability to endure longer periods without food. Specific health goals, whether for weight loss, detoxification, or other reasons, also guide the duration of the fast and should be considered before starting.

- *Monitoring*: Regular health monitoring is highly recommended during a water fast, especially for those undertaking extended periods without food. This includes tracking vital signs, energy levels, and any physical or mental changes. Consulting with healthcare professionals can provide additional support and ensure safety, helping to address any concerns that may arise during the fasting process.

3. **Intermittent Fasting**
    - ***Duration***: Flexible fasting periods can vary significantly, generally ranging from 12 to 48 hours. These periods can be repeated regularly, allowing individuals to choose a schedule that fits their lifestyle and needs, which can enhance adherence over time.

    - ***Sustainability***: This approach is often regarded as a long-term, sustainable lifestyle choice. It allows individuals to integrate fasting into their daily routines seamlessly, promoting a balanced relationship with food without the extreme deprivation associated with more rigid fasting types. This flexibility helps prevent feelings of restriction, making it easier to maintain in the long run.

    - ***Approach***: Among the popular methods, the 16:8 approach stands out, where individuals fast for 16 hours and eat during an 8-hour window, often skipping breakfast or dinner. Other variations, such as the 5:2 method, encourage normal eating five days a week, with caloric restriction limited to two non-consecutive days. This diversity in methods enables people to select an approach that best suits their preferences and daily rhythms, making fasting more attainable.

- ***Integration***: One of the significant advantages of this style of fasting is its versatility. It can be easily tailored to fit individual schedules and personal preferences, whether someone is a busy professional, a stay-at-home parent, or a student. This accessibility makes it an attractive option for most people who are looking to incorporate fasting into their lifestyle without the stress of rigid rules or complex meal planning.

Each fasting type offers distinct experiences and benefits, with dry fasting being the most intense, water fasting allowing for extended periods, and intermittent fasting providing a more adaptable and sustainable approach. Understanding the nuances of each can help individuals choose the method that best aligns with their health goals and lifestyle.

Outcomes and Experiences

- ***Dry Fasting***: Practitioners often report a heightened sense of mental clarity and rapid weight loss due to the body's shift into a state of ketosis, where it begins to burn fat for energy. However, it can be physically demanding, leading to symptoms such as fatigue and dehydration, and should be approached with caution, especially for those with pre-existing health conditions.

- ***Water Fasting***: Many individuals experience significant detoxification benefits and weight loss, as the body gets a chance to cleanse itself from toxins. Along with these advantages, participants may also encounter potential hunger pangs and fluctuations in energy levels, which can make the fasting experience challenging, especially in the initial days.

- ***Intermittent Fasting***: Users frequently note improved focus and cognitive function, making it easier to complete tasks throughout the day. This method often leads to easier weight management, as it promotes a natural reduction in calorie intake, along with increased energy levels during fasting periods. Additionally, it comes with less stringent dietary restrictions, allowing for more flexibility in food choices compared to other fasting methods.

Each fasting type offers unique benefits and challenges. Individuals should consider their health goals, lifestyle, and how each method aligns with their needs before choosing a fasting practice. Consulting with a healthcare professional is advised, especially for those considering more intensive fasting methods like dry fasting.

Pros and Cons of Dry Fasting

While dry fasting offers apparent benefits, such as rapid weight loss and detoxification, it also poses potential risks. The extreme nature of this method should be approached with caution and only practiced under the supervision of a healthcare professional. Here are some pros and cons to consider:

Pros

However, beyond the health benefits, dry fasting offers several practical advantages that make it an appealing choice for many. The following are some of the most notable pros of dry fasting:

1. ***Simplicity***: One of the most appealing aspects of this approach is its simplicity. There's no need for extensive meal planning or complicated dietary adjustments, making it straightforward to implement for anyone, regardless of their culinary skills or experience.
2. ***Time-Saving***: This method significantly reduces the time spent on preparing and consuming meals. By cutting out meal prep and dining, individuals can allocate that time to other activities they enjoy, pursue personal interests, or simply take a moment for reflection and mindfulness.

3. ***Minimal Resources Required***: Another advantage is that it requires very few resources. There's no need for special ingredients, expensive supplements, or sophisticated kitchen equipment, which makes this approach accessible to a broader range of people, regardless of their financial situation or living conditions.
4. ***Focus on Discipline***: This practice not only aids in physical health but also encourages mental discipline and self-control. By removing the distractions associated with eating and drinking, individuals can enhance their focus on personal goals, work, or spiritual practices, fostering a sense of clarity and purpose.
5. ***Cultural and Spiritual Alignment***: Furthermore, this approach can easily align with certain cultural or religious practices that emphasize abstinence or fasting. Many cultures have traditions that support periods of fasting, and this method can seamlessly fit into those beliefs, providing both spiritual fulfillment and health benefits.

Cons

While dry fasting may offer various benefits, it's essential to consider the potential drawbacks before deciding if this method is right for you. Here are some cons to keep in mind:

1. *Nutrient Deficiencies*: With no intake of food or water during dry fasting, it may be challenging to meet daily nutrient requirements. This lack of essential vitamins and minerals can lead to deficiencies over time, potentially resulting in fatigue, weakened immunity, and other health issues that could affect daily functioning.
2. *Highly Restrictive*: The strict nature of dry fasting, which prohibits both food and liquid intake, may make it difficult for some individuals to follow and sustain long-term. Many people find it hard to adhere to such a rigorous regimen, especially those who have busy lifestyles or high physical demands that require regular nourishment and hydration.
3. *Potential for Overeating*: After a prolonged period of restriction, there is a significant risk of overeating once the fasting period ends. This can lead to a cycle of binge eating and might offset any potential weight loss benefits gained during the fasting phase, leading to feelings of guilt and frustration.
4. *Not Suitable for Everyone*: It's important to recognize that dry fasting may not be suitable for everyone, particularly individuals with pre-existing medical conditions or those taking certain medications. Conditions such as diabetes, kidney disease, or heart issues can be exacerbated by dehydration and fasting. Therefore, it's crucial to consult a healthcare

professional before trying this method to ensure it aligns with one's health needs and lifestyle.

Overall, dry fasting can be an effective tool for weight loss and other potential health benefits. Still, it's essential to approach it with caution and proper knowledge to ensure safety and maximize its potential benefits.

Additionally, incorporating occasional dry fasts into a well-balanced diet and lifestyle may be a more sustainable approach than prolonged or frequent periods of restriction. As always, listen to your body and make informed decisions about what works best for you. So, consider all the pros and cons before starting this practice.

Risk and Precautions

Dry fasting, which involves abstaining from both food and water for a set period, is a practice that comes with several health risks. Understanding these risks and taking necessary precautions is crucial for anyone considering this approach.

Health Risks of Dry Fasting

1. *Dehydration*: Without water intake, the risk of dehydration is significant. Dehydration can lead to symptoms such as dizziness, confusion, decreased urine output, and severe headaches.
2. *Nutrient Deficiency*: Abstaining from both food and water can lead to a rapid decline in essential nutrients

and electrolytes, which may compromise bodily functions.
3. ***Kidney Strain***: The lack of water intake puts extra strain on the kidneys, increasing the risk of kidney stones and other kidney-related issues.
4. ***Organ Stress***: Vital organs, including the liver and heart, may experience increased stress as they work harder to maintain balance without the support of food and water.
5. ***Lack of Scientific Support***: There is limited scientific evidence supporting the benefits of dry fasting, and many health professionals express concern over its safety.

Importance of Consulting Healthcare Professionals

Before attempting dry fasting, it is critical to consult with healthcare professionals. They can provide personalized advice based on individual health conditions, ensuring the safety and appropriateness of such a fasting method.

Recommendations for those who should AVOID dry fasting

- ***Pregnant Women***: During pregnancy, the nutritional needs of women are significantly heightened due to the demands of both the mother and the developing fetus. This makes dry fasting particularly risky, as it can lead to dehydration and nutrient deficiencies that could negatively impact both maternal and fetal health.

- ***Individuals with Chronic Illnesses***: For those with chronic conditions like diabetes, cardiovascular diseases, or renal issues, consistent management of diet and hydration is crucial for maintaining health and preventing complications. Dry fasting can disrupt this delicate balance, making it unsafe and potentially harmful.
- ***Those on Medication***: Many medications require food or water for proper absorption into the body. Without adequate intake, the effectiveness of these medications can be compromised, and patients may also experience irritation to the stomach lining, leading to discomfort or adverse effects. It's essential for individuals on medication to prioritize their dietary needs to ensure optimal health outcomes.

Strategies to minimize risks

For those who still choose to proceed with dry fasting, the following strategies can help minimize potential risks:

- ***Gradual Adaptation***: Start with shorter periods of abstention from food and beverages to allow your body to adjust gradually to the changes. This approach helps minimize discomfort and prepares your system for longer fasting durations in the future, making the transition smoother and more manageable.
- ***Monitor Hydration Levels***: It's crucial to pay close attention to signs of dehydration during fasting, such

as dry mouth, fatigue, dizziness, and dark urine. If you notice any of these symptoms, be ready to break the fast to rehydrate properly. Staying aware of how your body feels can help you maintain your well-being throughout the fasting period.

- ***Balanced Diet Before and After***: Make sure to meet your nutritional needs with a well-rounded diet before starting the fast. Incorporate a variety of food groups, focusing on whole grains, lean proteins, fruits, and vegetables. After the fast, prioritize rehydration and nutrient replenishment immediately. Consuming a balanced meal that includes electrolytes and essential vitamins will help your body recover effectively and restore energy levels.

Dry fasting carries significant risks and should be approached with caution. Comprehensive planning and professional guidance are essential to ensure health and safety.

Potential Benefits of Dry Fasting

Dry fasting, although challenging, offers a myriad of potential benefits that span physical, mental, emotional, spiritual, and cultural dimensions. This chapter explores these benefits in detail, offering insights into how dry fasting can transform various aspects of life.

Physical Health Benefits

1. **Weight Loss**

    One of the most sought-after benefits of dry fasting is weight loss. The absence of both food and water intake compels the body to enter a state of ketosis more rapidly, where fat stores are utilized as the primary energy source. This accelerated fat metabolism can result in significant weight loss, especially for those seeking quick, short-term results. Additionally, dry fasting can lead to a reduction in overall calorie intake due to the absence of eating opportunities, further supporting weight loss goals.

2. **Detoxification**

   Dry fasting enhances the body's natural detoxification processes. During a fast, the body shifts its energy from digestion to maintenance and repair, initiating processes like autophagy. This cellular cleansing mechanism allows the body to break down and recycle damaged cells and proteins, effectively eliminating toxins and promoting healthier cell function. The intensified recycling and repair processes during dry fasting can lead to a rejuvenated and detoxified system.

3. **Improved Metabolism**

   Engaging in dry fasting can enhance metabolic health by improving insulin sensitivity and glucose metabolism. The reduction in insulin levels during fasting periods encourages the body to become more efficient in using glucose, potentially lowering the risk of developing insulin resistance and type 2 diabetes. Furthermore, the metabolic shift towards ketone utilization can lead to improved energy efficiency and metabolic flexibility.

Mental and Emotional Benefits

1. **Enhanced Mental Clarity**

   Many practitioners of dry fasting report heightened mental clarity and focus. The metabolic state of ketosis, induced more rapidly during dry fasting, provides the brain with a stable alternative energy source in the form of ketones. This can enhance cognitive function, improve concentration, and foster a sense of mental alertness. Additionally, the practice of fasting often requires a mindful approach, which can lead to increased awareness and mental presence.

2. **Emotional Resilience**

   The discipline and self-control required during dry fasting can cultivate emotional resilience. As the body adapts to the absence of food and water, individuals often experience a surge in willpower and emotional strength. This resilience can translate to greater emotional stability and a better ability to cope with stress and challenges in everyday life. The practice of fasting may also encourage introspection and self-reflection, leading to personal growth and emotional balance.

3. **Spiritual and Cultural Significance**

Dry fasting holds profound spiritual and cultural significance across various traditions. In many religions, such as Islam and Christianity, fasting is a common practice used to purify the soul, enhance spiritual awareness, and cultivate a closer connection to the divine. The act of abstaining from worldly needs is seen as a form of devotion, fostering humility and spiritual reflection.

Culturally, dry fasting is often integral to rituals and ceremonies, symbolizing renewal and purification. It is a time for individuals to reconnect with their spiritual beliefs and engage in communal practices that strengthen cultural identity and unity.

In summary, dry fasting offers a diverse range of benefits that extend beyond physical health, touching on mental clarity, emotional fortitude, and spiritual enrichment. Understanding these potential benefits can empower individuals to approach dry fasting with informed intentions, aligning their fasting practice with personal and cultural goals.

5-Step Plan to Getting Started with Dry Fasting

Starting a new fasting method can be daunting, but with proper preparation and guidance, dry fasting can be an effective and sustainable practice. Here is a 5-step plan to help you get started:

Step 1: Research and Education about Dry Fasting

Before diving into dry fasting, it's essential to arm yourself with the knowledge to ensure a safe and effective experience. Start by understanding what dry fasting entails—abstaining from both food and water for a set period, which can range from several hours to multiple days, depending on your goals and experience level. This practice is believed to promote various health benefits, but it's crucial to approach it with caution.

Explore a variety of resources such as comprehensive books, reputable articles, and expert opinions to gather a well-rounded understanding of the practice. Look for information from nutritionists and medical professionals who specialize in fasting or dietary practices. Consider the different types of dry fasting, such as soft dry fasting, where contact with water is allowed for activities like washing hands or showering, and hard dry fasting, which prohibits any contact with water at all, even during cleansing activities.

Familiarize yourself with the potential benefits that enthusiasts often highlight, such as weight loss, enhanced mental clarity, and detoxification of the body, which may lead to improved overall health. However, it's equally important to understand the associated risks. Dehydration, nutrient deficiencies, and possible adverse reactions can occur, especially if one is not adequately prepared or has pre-existing health conditions.

By thoroughly researching and understanding both the benefits and risks of dry fasting, you'll be better equipped to evaluate whether it aligns with your health goals and lifestyle. Consulting with a healthcare provider before starting any fasting regimen is also advisable to ensure it is appropriate for your individual health needs.

Step 2: Consult with a Healthcare Provider for Personalized Advice

Embarking on a dry fasting journey requires careful consideration and professional guidance. Consulting with a healthcare provider is a critical step to ensure your safety and well-being throughout the process. Here's why professional advice is indispensable and what to expect during a consultation.

Why Consulting a Healthcare Provider is Crucial

Dry fasting can have profound effects on your body, making it essential to seek medical advice before starting. A healthcare provider can offer personalized insights based on your unique health profile, ensuring that your fasting practice does not compromise your overall health. They can help you understand the risks and determine if dry fasting aligns with your physical condition.

Who Should Particularly Seek Advice

Certain individuals should prioritize consulting a healthcare professional before attempting dry fasting:

- ***Individuals with Chronic Health Issues***: Those with conditions such as diabetes, heart disease, or kidney problems may face heightened risks during dry fasting. This is due to the potential for complications, such as fluctuations in blood sugar levels or electrolyte imbalances. Therefore, they require tailored advice from healthcare professionals to ensure their safety and well-being during fasting periods.

- ***People Taking Medications***: Medication interactions can occur when food and water intake are restricted, which may lead to reduced effectiveness of medications or increased side effects. For instance, some medications require food for optimal absorption. This makes professional guidance essential to help individuals navigate their medication schedules and avoid any adverse effects that could arise from fasting.

- ***Pregnant or Breastfeeding Women***: Nutritional needs significantly increase during pregnancy and breastfeeding to support both maternal health and the development of the baby. Fasting might not be safe or advisable during these critical periods, as it can lead to nutrient deficiencies or dehydration. Therefore, medical supervision is vital to ensure that both the mother and child receive adequate nutrition.

- ***Elderly Individuals***: Older adults often face unique health challenges, including potential frailty and the presence of multiple chronic conditions. Dry fasting can put additional stress on their bodies, leading to dehydration or adverse health outcomes. For this reason, they should seek thorough medical evaluation and personalized advice from healthcare providers before engaging in any fasting regimen to ensure their safety and health are prioritized.

Aspects of Health Assessed by Healthcare Providers

During your consultation, healthcare providers will assess various health aspects to determine the suitability of dry fasting:

- ***Current Health Status***: A comprehensive evaluation of your overall health and any existing medical conditions will be conducted to thoroughly understand potential risks. This assessment may include reviewing your medical history, conducting physical examinations, and possibly running necessary laboratory tests to ensure a clear picture of your current health.

- ***Nutritional Needs***: Your nutritional requirements will be carefully analyzed to ensure they are not compromised during fasting. This analysis will take into account your dietary preferences, any food allergies you may have, and specific macro and micronutrient needs to maintain optimal health while fasting.

- ***Hydration Levels***: Proper hydration is critical for overall health and well-being. Your ability to maintain safe hydration levels during dry fasting will be assessed through various methods, including evaluating your fluid intake habits and monitoring your body's responses to fasting to prevent dehydration.

- ***Physical Fitness***: Your general physical fitness and resilience will be evaluated to determine how well your body might cope with fasting. This assessment may include measuring your cardiovascular endurance, strength levels, and flexibility, as well as discussing your typical physical activity levels and any exercise routines you currently follow, helping to tailor a fasting plan that suits your fitness level.

The Importance of Professional Guidance

By seeking professional advice, you gain access to expert recommendations that are vital for a safe and effective fasting experience:

- ***Personalized Guidance***: Healthcare providers can offer customized fasting plans tailored to your individual health needs and lifestyle, or suggest safer alternatives that better suit your unique health status. This personalized approach ensures that your fasting experience is both effective and safe, taking into account factors such as medical history, current medications, and dietary preferences.

- ***Risk Mitigation***: They can help you understand the potential complications that may arise during fasting and provide strategies for managing them effectively.

This knowledge ensures that you embark on your fasting journey with confidence, equipped with the tools to address any challenges that might come up along the way, thereby minimizing risks to your health.

- ***Long-term Health Considerations***: Professional advice can assist you in aligning your fasting practices with your long-term health goals. By working closely with healthcare providers, you can make necessary adjustments to your fasting regimen that support your overall well-being, ensuring that your approach not only fits your immediate goals but also contributes positively to your health in the years to come.

Taking these steps ensures that you are fully informed and prepared for the possible challenges of dry fasting, allowing you to pursue your health goals with the security and support of professional insight.

Step 3: Start with Shorter Fasting Periods and Gradually Increase Duration

Embarking on a dry fasting journey requires a strategic and gradual approach. This ensures that your body can adapt to the changes while minimizing potential risks. Here's a detailed guide on how to begin your dry fasting practice safely and effectively.

Benefits of Starting Small

Starting with shorter fasting periods is crucial for several reasons:

1. ***Minimized Risk***

    Starting with shorter fasting periods significantly reduces the risk of adverse effects. Longer fasting durations can lead to dehydration and nutrient deficiencies, as the body is deprived of essential fluids and nutrients for extended periods. By gradually easing into fasting, you allow your body to adjust to these new conditions without overwhelming it.

    This approach minimizes the potential for dizziness, fatigue, and other negative symptoms, ensuring a healthier and more sustainable fasting practice. It is especially important for individuals with health concerns or pre-existing conditions to minimize risks by consulting with healthcare professionals and starting with manageable fasting durations.

2. ***Enhanced Adaptation***

    The human body is remarkably adaptable, but it requires time to adjust to new routines, including fasting. Gradually increasing fasting durations helps the body become accustomed to the absence of food and water, enhancing its overall resilience and tolerance. This gradual adaptation allows the body's metabolic processes to adjust, optimizing fat utilization and energy production.

Over time, your body becomes more efficient at managing energy reserves, which can lead to improved physical performance, mental clarity, and overall well-being. By starting small, you give yourself the opportunity to build a solid foundation for longer fasting periods, reducing the likelihood of burnout or discouragement.

3. *Improved Monitoring*

One of the key benefits of beginning with shorter fasts is the ability to closely monitor your physical and mental responses. This initial phase provides an opportunity to track how your body reacts to fasting, enabling you to identify any issues early on. Monitoring symptoms such as changes in energy levels, mood, and cognitive function is critical for making informed decisions about your fasting practice.

This self-awareness allows for timely adjustments, such as modifying fasting durations or increasing hydration and nutritional intake, to enhance overall safety and effectiveness. Developing a keen understanding of your body's signals is an invaluable skill that will support you throughout your fasting journey.

Transitioning from Intermittent Fasting to Dry Fasting

To ease into dry fasting, consider starting with intermittent fasting methods that include water intake:

Begin with Intermittent Fasting

Starting with intermittent fasting, particularly the 16:8 method, is a practical and effective way to ease into fasting and become familiar with extended fasting periods. This approach involves fasting for 16 hours each day and eating during an 8-hour window. It allows individuals to reap the benefits of fasting without the intensity of longer fasting periods.

Understanding the 16:8 Method

Fasting Period: During your fasting period, it's important to consume water, tea, coffee, or other non-caloric drinks to stay hydrated and help curb hunger. Staying hydrated can also aid in maintaining your energy levels throughout the day.

- Structure: The fasting approach involves fasting for a total of 16 hours and eating within an 8-hour window. This method allows your body to rest from constant digestion, which can lead to various health benefits, including improved metabolism and enhanced focus.

- Example Schedule: You can choose to eat between 12 p.m. and 8 p.m., allowing for lunch and dinner during this timeframe. Consequently, you'll fast from 8pm until 12 p.m. the next day. This means skipping breakfast, which can be a great way to start your day with a clean slate and a focus on productivity.

Benefits of the 16:8 Method

- Calorie Control: Limiting the hours during which you can eat, this approach can lead to a natural reduction in overall calorie intake. This restriction helps individuals become more mindful of their eating habits and may contribute to weight management over time.

- Metabolic Health: This practice supports digestion by giving the body scheduled breaks from processing food. During these fasting periods, the body can focus on repairing cells, balancing hormones, and improving metabolic functions, promoting overall health.

- Energy and Clarity: Many people report enhanced energy levels and improved mental clarity as a result of optimizing energy use. By allowing the body to utilize stored fat for fuel during fasting, individuals often experience sustained energy throughout the day and sharper focus, helping them to be more productive in their daily tasks.

Implementing the 16:8 Approach

Intermittent fasting can be a powerful tool for health and wellness when approached with careful planning and consideration. Here is a detailed guide to help you effectively integrate intermittent fasting into your lifestyle by choosing the right eating window, maintaining consistency, and focusing on balanced meals.

1. <u>Choose Your Window: Pick an 8-hour Period That Suits Your Lifestyle</u>

   Selecting the ideal 8-hour eating window is crucial for aligning intermittent fasting with your daily routine. Consider the following tips to find a schedule that works best for you:

   - *Assess Your Daily Schedule*: Identify when you naturally feel hungry and energetic. For some, a morning to early afternoon window (e.g., 9 AM to 5 PM) aligns with their work schedule and energy peaks. Others might prefer a noon to evening window (e.g., 12 PM to 8 PM) to accommodate late dinners with family or social gatherings.

   - *Consider Work and Social Commitments*: Choose a window that fits your professional and personal obligations. If you often have lunch meetings or dinner plans, adjust your window to accommodate these without feeling restricted.

- *Experiment and Adjust*: It might take some trial and error to find what suits you best. Start with a window that seems promising and adjust based on how your body responds and how well it fits into your lifestyle.

2. **<u>Consistency: Stick to the Same Eating Schedule Daily</u>**

Consistency is key to reaping the full benefits of intermittent fasting. Here's how to maintain a steady schedule:

- *Set Reminders*: Use alarms or calendar notifications to remind you of your eating and fasting periods. Consistency will become easier as it becomes part of your routine.

- *Stay Flexible Yet Committed*: Life can be unpredictable, so allow yourself some flexibility. If you need to adjust your window occasionally, do so without stress, but aim to return to your regular schedule promptly.

- *Monitor Progress*: Keep a journal to track how you feel, your energy levels, and any changes in weight or wellness. This feedback can motivate you to maintain consistency.

3. *Balanced Meals: Focus on Nutrient-Rich Meals to Sustain Energy Levels*

What you eat during your eating window is just as important as when you eat. Ensure your meals are balanced and nutritious:

- *Prioritize Nutrient-Dense Foods*: Fill your plate with a variety of fruits, vegetables, lean proteins, whole grains, and healthy fats. These foods provide sustained energy and essential nutrients needed for overall health.

- *Plan Your Meals*: Preparing meals in advance can help ensure you have healthy options readily available, reducing the temptation to grab fast or processed foods.

- *Stay Hydrated*: Drink plenty of water throughout the day to support digestion and metabolism. Herbal teas and black coffee are also good options if you need a change from water.

- *Listen to Your Body*: Pay attention to hunger cues and avoid overeating. Eating mindfully can help you enjoy your meals and prevent feelings of deprivation.

By carefully selecting your eating window, maintaining a consistent schedule, and focusing on balanced nutrition, you can maximize the benefits of intermittent fasting. These practices not only support weight management but also enhance energy levels and overall well-being.

Potential Challenges and Tips for Success

- Initial Adjustments: As your body begins to adapt to the new routine, you may experience initial feelings of hunger or low energy. This is a normal part of the adjustment period, and it's important to give your body time to acclimate to the changes. Be patient with yourself, as these feelings often diminish as your body adjusts.

- Stay Hydrated: It's crucial to drink plenty of fluids throughout the day. Staying well-hydrated can help you avoid confusing thirst with hunger, which is a common mistake. Aim for at least eight glasses of water daily, and consider incorporating herbal teas or flavored water to keep things interesting.

- Stay Active: Engaging in light exercise, such as walking, stretching, or yoga, can help manage hunger cues and boost your energy levels. Regular physical activity not only helps distract you from feelings of hunger but also supports your overall well-being and can enhance your mood during the adjustment phase.

The 16:8 method is a practical entry point into fasting, offering health benefits while fitting within your daily routine. With persistence, this approach can enhance well-being and prepare you for more extended fasting practices.

Move to Short Dry Fasts

After establishing a routine with intermittent fasting, you can gradually introduce short dry fasts as the next step in your fasting journey. This transition helps acclimate your body to periods without water intake, offering unique benefits.

Understanding Short Dry Fasts

- Definition: A dry fast, also known as absolute fasting, involves completely abstaining from both food and water for a specified period. This method is often practiced for spiritual or health reasons, pushing the body to adapt to a lack of hydration while still undergoing the benefits of fasting.

- Duration: The duration of a dry fast typically lasts between 6 to 8 hours, although some practitioners may extend this period. It is essential to listen to your body and ensure that you do not exceed limits that could cause discomfort or health risks.

- Difference: Unlike regular fasting, where only food is restricted and water is still consumed, dry fasting excludes any liquid intake. This exclusion intensifies the fasting experience, leading to quicker metabolic changes and potentially deeper detoxification. However, it's crucial to approach dry fasting with caution, as the lack of water can lead to dehydration if not done properly.

Benefits of Short Dry Fasts

- Enhanced Detoxification: The absence of water intake during dry fasting accelerates cellular repair and waste removal. This process allows the body to focus on eliminating toxins more efficiently, promoting overall health and rejuvenation at the cellular level.

- Increased Fat Burn: Without food or liquids, the body begins to tap into fat reserves more quickly, utilizing stored energy for fuel. This metabolic shift not only aids in weight loss but also encourages the body to become more efficient in burning fat as an energy source.

- Mental Clarity: Many individuals report experiencing heightened mental focus and clarity during dry fasting periods. This could be attributed to the body's shift towards ketosis, where it utilizes fat for energy, potentially leading to improved cognitive function and concentration.

Initiating Short Dry Fasts Safely

- Start Slowly: It's important to begin with shorter durations when starting a dry fast, such as 6 hours, to allow your body to adjust gradually. Over time, as you become more comfortable and your body adapts, you can increase the fasting duration to 8 hours. This gradual approach helps prevent any overwhelming feelings of hunger or discomfort as your body learns to cope with the absence of food and water.

- Timing: Consider starting your dry fast after a meal. This strategy can help sustain your energy levels during the initial hours of fasting, as your body will still be digesting food and converting it into energy. By doing this, you may find it easier to manage the transition into fasting and reduce feelings of fatigue.

- Preparation: Proper preparation is key to a successful dry fast. Make sure you are adequately hydrated before beginning, as this will help minimize discomfort during the fasting period. Drinking plenty of water in the days leading up to the fast can help ensure your body is well-hydrated, making the experience more manageable and less stressful on your system.

Potential Challenges and Tips for Success

- Hydration Concerns: Dehydration poses a significant risk during fasting, so it's crucial to be attentive to your body's signals. If you start feeling dizzy, fatigued, or excessively thirsty, don't hesitate to break the fast. Listening to your body's needs is essential for maintaining your health and well-being during this process.

- <u>Energy Levels</u>: Experiencing low energy levels is common in the initial stages of fasting, as your body adjusts to the lack of food intake. To manage this, it's a good idea to plan for ample rest periods or engage in light activities such as stretching or gentle walking. This approach can help you conserve energy and ease the transition.

- <u>Breaking the Fast</u>: When it's time to break your fast, it's important to do so gradually. Start by reintroducing water to rehydrate your body, followed by light foods such as broth or easily digestible fruits. This gradual reintroduction helps ease your digestive system back into action and minimizes any potential discomfort.

Transitioning to short dry fasts can deepen your fasting practice and amplify its benefits. With careful preparation and attention to your body's needs, you can safely explore this advanced fasting technique and enhance your overall well-being.

Gradually Increase Duration

As you become more accustomed to dry fasting, you can begin to extend the duration of your fasts. This gradual increase allows your body to adapt while maximizing the benefits associated with longer fasting periods.

The Importance of Listening to Your Body

- Body Signals: It's crucial to pay close attention to how your body feels during and after fasting. Note any signs of fatigue, hunger, or discomfort, as these can offer valuable insights into how your body is responding to the fast. Taking mental or physical notes can help you identify patterns over time.

- Adjustments: Be prepared to modify the fasting duration based on your energy levels, hydration status, and overall well-being. If you find yourself feeling excessively tired or dehydrated, consider shortening your fasting period or adjusting the timing to better suit your daily activities and lifestyle. Listening to your body and making thoughtful adjustments can enhance your fasting experience and support your health goals.

Safely Extending Fasting Duration

- Incremental Increase: Gradually extend your fasting period by adding a few hours at a time. This allows your body to adapt comfortably to the changes without overwhelming it. Start with small increments, such as 1-2 hours, and pay attention to how your body responds before increasing further.

- Monitor Closely: It's essential to keep a close eye on any physical or emotional changes during your fasting journey. Take notes on how you feel throughout the process, including energy levels, mood shifts, and hunger cues. This awareness will help you identify what works best for your body and ensure a safe and effective progression.

- Stay Hydrated Beforehand: Before starting each fast, make it a priority to hydrate adequately. Drinking plenty of water beforehand helps to prepare your body, reducing the risk of dehydration during longer fasting periods. Aim to consume fluids consistently in the hours leading up to your fast, so you enter the fasting phase feeling refreshed and ready.

Potential Benefits of Longer Dry Fasts

- Deeper Detoxification: Extended fasting can significantly enhance the body's natural detox processes, allowing for a more thorough elimination of toxins. During this time, the body can shift its focus from digestion to cellular repair and cleansing, promoting overall health and vitality.

- Improved Fat Metabolism: Spending more time without food and water encourages the body to switch its energy source, leading it to burn fat for fuel. This metabolic shift not only helps in weight loss but also improves energy levels, as stored fat becomes a more efficient source of energy when carbohydrates are limited.

- Enhanced Mental Resilience: Longer fasts can lead to improved mental clarity and focus. As the body adapts to the fasting state, individuals often report a heightened sense of awareness and cognitive function, fostering greater mental strength. This boost in mental resilience can help in various aspects of life, from decision-making to emotional stability during challenging situations.

Tips for Monitoring Health and Well-being

- Regular Check-ins: It's important to assess both your physical and mental well-being at regular intervals throughout the fasting period. Pay attention to how your body feels, any signs of fatigue or discomfort, and your overall mood to ensure you are managing your fast effectively.

- Break Gently: After completing your fast, take your time to gradually reintroduce water and light foods. Start with small sips of water, followed by easily digestible foods like broth or fruits, to help your digestive system adjust and prevent any discomfort that might arise from a sudden influx of heavier meals.

- <u>Rest and Relax</u>: Make sure to prioritize rest and engage in stress-reducing activities during your fasting journey, as extended fasting can place a significant physical demand on your body. Consider practices such as gentle yoga, meditation, or leisurely walks to help foster a sense of calm and rejuvenation.

By gradually increasing the duration of your dry fasts, you can explore deeper levels of fasting benefits while maintaining your health and safety. Always prioritize your body's signals and responses, and adjust your fasting routine accordingly to support your well-being.

Monitoring Physical and Mental Responses

Careful monitoring is essential to ensure your safety and well-being during dry fasting:

- *Physical Signals*: Be attentive to physical symptoms such as dizziness, fatigue, or headaches. These could indicate dehydration or nutrient deficiency and should not be ignored.

- *Mental Well-being*: Monitor your mental state, including mood changes, focus, and clarity. Notice how these aspects are affected and assess whether they improve or worsen over time.

- *Hydration Levels*: Although dry fasting involves abstaining from water, it is vital to stay aware of hydration levels. Should severe dehydration symptoms arise, consider ending the fast and consult a healthcare provider.

The Importance of a Gradual Approach

Taking a gradual approach to dry fasting is key to a successful and sustainable practice:

- *Listen to Your Body*: Always pay attention to your body's responses and never push beyond your comfort zone. Your body will signal when it needs nourishment and hydration.

- *Safety First*: Prioritize safety over fasting goals. If your body reacts negatively, scale back and consult a healthcare professional if necessary.

By carefully following these guidelines and adopting a gradual approach, you can explore the practice of dry fasting safely while maximizing its potential benefits.

Step 4: Implement Supportive Habits such as Proper Hydration Before and After Fasting

To ensure a safe and effective dry fasting experience, incorporating supportive habits, particularly focusing on hydration, is essential. Proper hydration before and after fasting can significantly impact the outcome and sustainability of your fasting journey. Here's a detailed guide on how to implement these supportive habits.

The Importance of Hydration

Hydration plays a crucial role in preparing your body for dry fasting and aiding recovery afterward:

- *Prevents Dehydration*: Ensuring proper hydration before entering a fasting period is crucial as it significantly mitigates the risk of dehydration during the fasting itself. This is especially important in dry fasting, where no water is consumed for an extended period. By starting off well-hydrated, your body can better cope with the absence of fluids, reducing the chance of experiencing symptoms like dizziness, fatigue, or headaches.

- *Supports Body Functions*: In addition to preventing dehydration, adequate water intake is vital for maintaining a wide range of essential bodily functions. Water plays a key role in circulation, helping transport nutrients and oxygen to cells, as well as in digestion, where it aids in breaking down food for better nutrient absorption. Furthermore, it is important for temperature regulation, allowing the body to maintain a stable internal environment, which is especially crucial during fasting when metabolic processes may fluctuate.

Pre-Fasting Hydration Tips

Preparing your body with effective hydration strategies before beginning your dry fast is key:

- *Increase Water Intake*: In the days leading up to your fast, gradually increase your water consumption to ensure optimal hydration levels. Aim to drink at least 8-10 glasses of water daily, and consider setting reminders throughout the day to help you stay on track. Staying well-hydrated not only prepares your body for the fast but also aids in digestion and overall well-being.

- *Consume Water-Rich Foods*: Incorporate foods with high water content, such as cucumbers, watermelon, and oranges, to boost hydration naturally. These foods not only keep you hydrated but also provide essential vitamins and minerals. For example, cucumbers are low in calories and high in fiber, making them a great snack option, while watermelon is refreshing and packed with antioxidants.

- *Balance Electrolytes*: Include electrolytes in your diet through foods like bananas, avocados, and spinach to maintain a proper balance of essential minerals. Electrolytes are crucial for regulating hydration, nerve function, and muscle contractions, especially during fasting. Consider adding a pinch of salt to your meals or enjoying coconut water for a natural electrolyte boost. This preparation will help your body function optimally during the fasting period.

Post-Fasting Rehydration Strategies

Rehydrating effectively after a dry fast is crucial to restore balance and avoid shocking your system:

- *Gradual Rehydration*: Begin rehydrating slowly to prevent overwhelming your body. Start with small sips of water and gradually increase the amount.

- *Include Electrolyte-Rich Drinks*: Use drinks like coconut water or specially formulated electrolyte beverages to replenish lost nutrients and support recovery.

- *Monitor Your Response*: Pay attention to how your body responds to rehydration, and adjust your intake as needed to ensure comfort and effectiveness.

The Role of Electrolytes

Electrolytes are vital to maintaining balance during and after dry fasting:

- *Prevent Imbalances*: Electrolytes help prevent imbalances that can occur from rapid fluid loss and are crucial for muscle function and nerve communication.

- ***Support Recovery***: Replenishing electrolytes post-fast can aid in recovery, ensuring your body returns to normal function more efficiently.

Developing Sustainable Habits

Incorporating these supportive habits can make your dry fasting practice more sustainable and enjoyable:

- ***Regular Hydration***: Make hydration a regular habit, not just a pre-fasting concern. Consistent hydration supports overall health and fasting readiness.

- ***Balanced Nutrition***: Focus on maintaining a balanced diet rich in essential nutrients and electrolytes to support your fasting goals.

By implementing these supportive hydration habits, you can enhance your dry fasting experience, reducing the risk of negative side effects and promoting better overall results.

Step 5: Monitor the Body's Response and Adjust the Approach as Necessary

Monitoring your body's response throughout the dry fasting process is crucial for ensuring safety and effectiveness. This involves being vigilant about physical and emotional cues and making necessary adjustments to your fasting routine.

Recognizing Signs that Require Attention

During and after dry fasting, it's important to be aware of signs that may indicate the need to pause or stop:

1. *Dizziness*: Feeling lightheaded can be a sign of dehydration or low blood pressure, both of which require immediate attention. This sensation may occur when the body lacks adequate fluids or nutrients, causing the blood pressure to drop and leading to inadequate blood flow to the brain. If this feeling persists, it's crucial to hydrate and seek medical advice.

2. *Extreme Fatigue*: Experiencing unusual levels of tiredness can indicate that your body is struggling to cope with the fasting conditions. This fatigue may stem from a lack of essential calories and nutrients, leaving you feeling drained and lethargic. It's important to listen to your body, and if extreme fatigue continues, consider adjusting your fasting approach or consulting a healthcare professional.

3. *Confusion*: Mental fog or confusion can be serious signs of electrolyte imbalance or dehydration. These symptoms can impair cognitive function, making it difficult to think clearly or focus. Electrolytes play a vital role in maintaining nerve and muscle function, so an imbalance can lead to significant issues. If you find

yourself confused or unable to concentrate, it's important to rehydrate and restore electrolyte levels promptly.

Being proactive about these symptoms can prevent potential health issues and ensure that your fasting practice remains safe.

Benefits of Keeping a Fasting Journal

A fasting journal is a valuable tool for tracking your experiences and responses during dry fasting:

- ***Track Physical Symptoms***: It's essential to document any physical changes you experience during your fasting journey. This includes monitoring energy levels, noting any headaches, or recognizing digestive issues. By keeping a detailed record, you can help identify patterns or recurring issues that may arise, allowing you to make informed decisions about your health and fasting practices.

- ***Monitor Emotional State***: Pay close attention to any changes in your mood or mental clarity throughout your fasting periods. Documenting these fluctuations will provide insight into how fasting affects your psychological well-being. Understanding the emotional aspects of fasting can help you navigate challenges and improve your overall experience.

- *Identify Trends*: Over time, your journal will become a valuable resource, revealing trends that can significantly inform adjustments to your fasting strategy. By analyzing these patterns, you can enhance both the safety and effectiveness of your fasting regimen, tailoring it to better suit your individual needs and lifestyle. This thoughtful approach can lead to more successful and sustainable fasting outcomes.

Adjusting the Fasting Approach Based on Observations

Using insights from your fasting journal and body signals, you can tailor your approach to better suit your needs:

- *Modify Duration*: If you notice that certain symptoms consistently arise during your fasting periods, it may be beneficial to shorten your fasting duration temporarily. This adjustment allows your body to gradually adapt to the changes and ensures that you can still reap the benefits of fasting without discomfort.

- *Alter Frequency*: If you find that your recovery takes longer than expected or if adverse effects such as fatigue or irritability persist, consider adjusting the frequency of your fasts. Finding the right balance can help you maintain your well-being while still pursuing your fasting goals.

- ***Incorporate Breaks***: Integrating rest periods or less intense fasting phases into your routine can be incredibly helpful. These breaks provide your body with the opportunity to recuperate, helping to prevent burnout and allowing you to maintain a healthy balance in your fasting practice. By listening to your body and incorporating these strategies, you can create a more sustainable and enjoyable fasting experience.

By diligently monitoring your body's response and maintaining a detailed record, you can make informed decisions about your fasting practice. This proactive approach ensures that your dry fasting experience remains both safe and beneficial, allowing you to achieve your health objectives effectively.

By following these steps, you can embark on your dry fasting journey with greater confidence and safety. Remember, the key to successful fasting is to proceed mindfully and prioritize your health above all else.

Conclusion

Congratulations on reaching the end of this comprehensive guide on dry fasting! Your curiosity and dedication to understanding this unique practice are commendable. Navigating through the realm of health and wellness requires an open mind and a cautious approach, and you've taken an important step by equipping yourself with knowledge.

Dry fasting, as you've learned, is a practice that involves abstaining from both food and water for a specific period. While some advocates claim potential benefits, such as detoxification and spiritual enhancement, it's crucial to approach these claims with a healthy dose of skepticism and an understanding of your body's needs. Every person is different, and what works for one might not be suitable for another.

Throughout this guide, you've explored various aspects of dry fasting—its potential benefits, the risks involved, and the historical and cultural contexts in which it exists. This knowledge empowers you to make informed decisions. Remember, your health should always be the top priority.

Before considering any fasting routine, consulting with healthcare professionals is vital. They can offer personalized advice based on your individual health profile, ensuring that any health practice you try is safe and appropriate.

It's important to recognize that dry fasting is not universally recommended and carries potential risks, especially for those with underlying health conditions. Dehydration, electrolyte imbalances, and other serious health issues can arise from improper fasting practices. These risks underscore the importance of professional guidance and monitoring if you decide to explore fasting further.

However, don't let this deter you from pursuing a path to wellness that resonates with you. There are numerous ways to enhance your health and vitality, each with its own set of benefits and considerations. Whether it's through balanced nutrition, regular exercise, mindfulness practices, or other types of fasting like intermittent fasting, it's about finding what aligns best with your personal lifestyle and health goals.

Your journey to wellness is deeply personal and ongoing. It's about understanding your body, honoring your needs, and making choices that foster your overall well-being. As you continue to explore various health and wellness practices, keep an open mind and a critical eye. Be willing to adapt and learn, and remember that the ultimate goal is to nurture a healthy and fulfilling life.

As a steward of your own health journey, you have the power to shape it in a way that benefits you the most. Engage with communities, seek diverse perspectives, and continue educating yourself. The world of health and wellness is vast and ever-evolving, offering endless opportunities for discovery and personal growth.

Thank you for investing your time in reading this guide. Your pursuit of knowledge is a testament to your commitment to health and self-improvement. We hope this guide has provided valuable insights and sparked thoughtful consideration about the role dry fasting might—or might not—play in your life.

Stay curious, stay informed, and most importantly, prioritize your well-being in all your endeavors. You are your best advocate and the most qualified person to decide what aligns with your health journey. May your path forward be filled with health, happiness, and continuous discovery.

FAQs

What is dry fasting?

Dry fasting is a practice where an individual abstains from both food and water for a set period. It is often pursued for spiritual, health, or detoxification purposes, though it is not scientifically validated as a safe or effective health practice for everyone.

What are the potential benefits of dry fasting?

Some proponents claim dry fasting may lead to benefits like detoxification, improved mental clarity, and spiritual growth. However, these claims lack substantial scientific backing, and the practice's safety and efficacy remain subjects of debate among health experts.

What are the risks associated with dry fasting?

Risks of dry fasting include dehydration, electrolyte imbalances, and potential kidney damage. It can also exacerbate underlying health conditions, making it crucial to approach this practice with caution and professional guidance.

How long can a person safely dry fast?

The duration of a dry fast can vary, but even short periods without water can be dangerous. It is essential to consult with healthcare professionals to assess any risks based on individual health conditions before attempting a dry fast.

How should one prepare for a dry fast?

Proper preparation for dry fasting involves gradually reducing food and water intake, ensuring adequate hydration beforehand, and planning for rest and monitoring during the fast. Consultation with a healthcare provider is strongly advised to tailor the preparation process to individual needs.

Is dry fasting safe for everyone?

Dry fasting is not safe for everyone. Individuals with chronic health conditions, pregnant or breastfeeding women, children, and the elderly should avoid dry fasting. It is critical to consult with a healthcare professional to determine if dry fasting is appropriate and safe for you.

Who should avoid dry fasting?

Those with health conditions such as diabetes, heart disease, kidney problems, or those who are pregnant or breastfeeding should avoid dry fasting. Always seek medical advice before considering dry fasting to ensure it does not pose undue risks to your health.

References and Helpful Links

Nunez, K. (2019, October 30). Everything you want to know about dry fasting. Healthline.
https://www.healthline.com/health/food-nutrition/dry-fasting

Koppold-Liebscher, D. A., Klatte, C., Demmrich, S., Schwarz, J., Kandil, F. I., Steckhan, N., Ring, R., Kessler, C. S., Jeitler, M., Koller, B., Ananthasubramaniam, B., Eisenmann, C., Mähler, A., Boschmann, M., Kramer, A., & Michalsen, A. (2021). Effects of daytime dry fasting on hydration, glucose metabolism and circadian phase: a prospective exploratory cohort study in Bahá'í volunteers. Frontiers in Nutrition, 8.
https://doi.org/10.3389/fnut.2021.662310

Bryant, J. (2024, April 26). Fasting & Socialising: Turning Challenges into Opportunities.
https://www.linkedin.com/pulse/fasting-socialising-turning-challenges-opportunities-john-bryant-k3yte

Clinic, C. (2024, August 1). Dry fasting: Why you should avoid it. Cleveland Clinic.
https://health.clevelandclinic.org/dry-fasting#:~:text=Fans%20claim%20dry%20fasting%20benefits,reducing%20inflammation%20and%20delaying%20aging.

Trabelsi, K., Ammar, A., Boujelbane, M. A., Puce, L., Garbarino, S., Scoditti, E., Boukhris, O., Khanfir, S., Clark, C. C. T., Glenn, J. M., Alhaj, O. A., Jahrami, H., Chtourou, H., & Bragazzi, N. L. (2022).

bloReligious fasting and its impacts on individual, public, and planetary health: Fasting as a "religious health asset" for a healthier, more equitable, and sustainable society. Frontiers in Nutrition, 9. https://doi.org/10.3389/fnut.2022.1036496

Chiu, M. (2023, January 4). Dawn-to-dusk dry fasting leads to health benefits in the study of immune cells. Baylor College of Medicine. https://www.bcm.edu/news/dawn-to-dusk-dry-fasting-leads-to-health-benefits-in-the-study-of-immune-cells

Yamut, T. J., RN. (2023, March 20). Dry Fasting: How it Works, Benefits, Risks, and Safety. Perfect Keto. https://perfectketo.com/dry-fasting/#:~:text=Because%20dry%20fasting%20doesn't,most%20at%20risk%20of%20dehydration.

www.ingramcontent.com/pod-product-compliance
Lightning Source LLC
LaVergne TN
LVHW012034060526
838201LV00061B/4610